Navigating the Skies of Success

A Collegiate Aviator's Guide to Mental Wellness

Reyné O'Shaughnessy

Legal and Copyright

Copyright © Reyné O'Shaughnessy

All rights reserved. No part of this publication may be reproduced, distributed, or transmitted in any form or by any means, including photocopying, recording, or other electronic or mechanical methods, without the prior written permission of the publisher, except in the case of brief quotations embodied in critical reviews and certain other noncommercial uses permitted by copyright law.

Published in the United States by
Create Your Authority Press
#1272 18 Folly Rd. Ste B9
Charleston, SC 29407
www.CreateYourAuthorityPress.com

Ordering Information:
Special discounts are available on quantity purchases by corporations, associations, and others. For details, contact the Reyné O'Shaughnessy at:.

info@piloting2wellbeing.com
www.Piloting2Wellbeing.com

Printed in the United States of America

Contents

Dedication	V
Preface	VI
Foreword	XIV
1. The Importance of Mental Health in Aviation	1
2. Mental Health Awareness in Aviation	9
3. Understanding Stressors in Collegiate Pilots	22
4. Nurturing Mental Wellness for Optimal Pilot Performance	40
5. The Impact of Mental Health on Pilot Performance	50
6. Building Resilience in Collegiate Pilots	60
7. Prevention and Habits for a Healthier Cockpit	67

8. Awakening the Aviator Within ~ The How-To Guide — 72

9. The Role of Support Systems — 79

10. Q&A Session — 87

11. Making Mental Health a Priority in Aviation — 94

To

John A Hauser, whose dedicated passion for aviation was met with his strong desire to help others.

He is always in our hearts.

Preface

> "Aviation is proof that given the will, we have the capacity to achieve the impossible."
> —Eddie Rickenbacker

Welcome aboard, fellow aviators, to a journey that will take you soaring through the skies of knowledge and experience. As an experienced commercial pilot with 47 years in the airline industry and over 35 years as a veteran jet pilot, I have had the privilege of flying some of the most iconic aircraft, totaling over 10,000 hours in the cockpit.

I am honored to bring you *Navigating the Skies of Success: A Collegiate Aviator's Guide to Mental Wellness.*

This book is the culmination of a lifelong passion for aviation and a burning desire to empower the next generation of aviators. My journey in aviation began with the wonder and curiosity of a young pilot, and with each flight, I yearned for knowledge and guidance that could have made my path smoother. It is from this very longing that I set out to make my education and experience as an aviator accessible to collegiate students.

Throughout these pages, you will find a treasure trove of wisdom, advice, and insights garnered from years of navigating the skies and encountering the highs and lows of this extraordinary profession. Each chapter is carefully crafted to equip you with the tools you need to not only succeed as a collegiate aviation student but also to thrive in your future career.

The journey begins with a crucial topic often overlooked – health and mental wellness because it is an integral part of safety. Safety to you, and to our skies.

In the Talking Segment: "The Importance of Mental Wellness in Aviation," we will explore the significance of mental wellness in aviation. As collegiate pilots, it is vital to understand how our mental state directly influences our performance in the cockpit. We will delve into eye-opening studies and research that highlight the undeniable link between mental health and aviation performance.

Chapter 1: "Elevating Aviation Performance through Mental Health" This opening chapter emphasizes the critical role of mental wellness in aviation, positioning it as an equal partner to technical skills in piloting. It vividly illustrates how mental health significantly influences communication, decision-making, reaction time, situational awareness, and overall performance in aviation. The chapter explores Threat and Error Management (TEM), highlighting how mentally resilient pilots are better equipped to identify and address threats and errors. It also acknowledges the unique challenges faced by collegiate aviators, emphasizing the importance of personal and professional growth in their aviation journey.

Chapter 2: "Resilience: The Key to Aviation Success" Chapter two focuses on resilience and what it means in aviation. It's an adaptable skill that enables individuals to rebound from setbacks and adapt to changing circumstances. It underscores the critical role of coping strategies, including stress management, mindfulness practices, peer and mentor support, and rejuvenating activities.

But there's more: Competency and Confidence are the foundation for resilience in aviation, and you'll learn what fuels each. The chapter advocates for an open dialogue culture regarding mental wellness and underscores the value of sharing personal experiences to foster relatability and solidarity within the aviation community.

Chapter 3: "Navigating the Skies of Stress: Understanding Collegiate Pilots" In this chapter, readers explore the common stressors affecting collegiate aviation students, including academic pressures, financial stress, performance anxiety, and the impact of social media. The chapter provides practical strategies for managing these stressors, such as effective time management, mindfulness techniques, stress reduction methods, judicious social media use, and building supportive relationships. Personal anecdotes and real-life stories vividly illustrate the significance of these strategies in the challenging world of aviation.

Chapter 4: "The Nexus of Mental Wellness and Aviation Safety" The book's preface welcomes budding aviation professionals, unveiling the deep connection between mental wellness and aviation safety. It underscores the vital role of mental health in ensuring job performance and the safety of flight operations. The preface emphasizes the urgency of prioritizing mental wellness on the path to becoming skilled and responsible aviators, setting the stage for the subsequent chapters that explore the profound relationship between mental health and pilot performance.

Chapter 5: "Performance and Safety: The Mental Wellness Connection" This preface delves into the inherent link between job performance and safety in aviation. It highlights the solemn responsibility of aviators for the safety of passengers, crew members, and aircraft. The preface introduces eye-opening studies and research, demonstrating how mental health permeates various aspects of pilot performance, including communication, technical skills, decision-making, and situational awareness. It emphasizes the need to address mental health to enhance pilot performance and elevate aviation safety.

In **Chapter 6:** "Building Resilience in Collegiate Pilots," we will uncover strategies to cultivate mental resilience during pilot training and beyond. As future aviators, resilience is the cornerstone of navigating the challenges that come our way. By embracing a growth mindset and practicing mindfulness, we can develop the fortitude needed to conquer obstacles and emerge stronger from setbacks.

Chapter 7: "Prevention and Habits for a Healthier Cockpit" will introduce proactive measures to promote a healthier flight deck environment. We will explore the power of teamwork and communication among crew members and discuss habits that enhance mental clarity, focus, and overall well-being during flights.

The journey continues with **Chapter 8**: "Awakening the Aviator Within - The How-To Guide." In the fast-paced world of aviation, self-awareness and mindfulness are powerful tools that can positively impact our wellness and performance. By recognizing and understanding our emotions, thoughts, and actions and staying fully present in the moment, we can make more informed decisions and forge a deeper connection to the flight experience.

Chapter 9: "The Role of Support Systems" highlights the importance of having a strong support system during training and beyond. We will discuss the benefits of mentorship, coaching, peer support, and seeking professional help when needed. Remember, you are not alone on this aviation adventure, and embracing support systems will fuel your growth and success. For the intent of this book, wellbeing and wellness will be used interchangeably.

Finally, we arrive at **Chapter 10:** "Q&A Session," where you will find often-asked questions about health and mental well-being in aviation, building resilience, or any other topic we've discussed. The questions and discussions are invaluable, and I am here to support you in every way I can.

In closing, I extend my deepest gratitude for embarking on this journey with me. As you absorb the knowledge within these pages, I hope you will find inspiration, encouragement, and a renewed sense of passion for aviation. May this book serve as a compass, guiding you toward a fulfilling and prosperous aviation career.

Together, let us soar to new heights, for the sky is limitless, and the possibilities are boundless.

May your dreams take flight, and may you find fulfillment in the captivating world of aviation.

Blue skies and safe flights always,

Captain O

Foreword

For collegiate flight training students, the art of balancing academic commitments, while navigating the complex skies of flight training can be daunting. Stress, anxiety, and depression can hinder a student's ability to complete collegiate flight training. Anxiety and stress are intrinsic to flight training and therefore cannot be eliminated.

These stressors can negatively affect the flight student's mental health and decrease the likelihood of completing their flight training. This is where Captain (ret.) Reyne O'Shaughnessy, known as Captain O, steps in to guide collegiate flight training students through these turbulent times and the beginning of solutions.

Navigating the Skies of Success explores the four fundamental Navigational Points of pilot wellness beginning with: sleep, nutrition, exercise, and relaxation.

As you read this book, you will gain a greater understanding of the essentials that will keep you healthy and flying healthily. *Navigating the Skies of Success* is a toolkit with simple, yet powerful solutions tailored just for the collegiate aviator. Captain O provides tips at the end of the chapters that allow you to roll up your sleeves and dive right in. There are also "notes" sections that allow you to record your thoughts on paper, as well as your dreams and aspirations. Much has been written about pilot mental wellness; however, *Navigating the Skies of Success* is an active journey with tips and signposts that will guide you to smoother skies. What distinguishes this book is its simplicity. Captain O provides you with tools that are straightforward and customized for collegiate aviators.

This is your blueprint for a successful journey through collegiate flight training and beyond. The knowledge you gain will be your compass in the vast skies of your professional aviation career, all while prioritizing your mental wellness.

More importantly, this book provides encouragement and instills a sense of hope to those that are struggling with mental wellness. The journey through collegiate aviation is electrifying, complex and, at times, overwhelming. The recurring theme Captain O weaves into this book is that "you are not alone." Slowly the stigma surrounding mental wellness is being eroded within the aviation industry, and collegiate aviators no longer need to struggle in silence. Captain O is helping to change the culture of collegiate aviation to promote acceptance, openness, and understanding.

Captain O is a seasoned aviator with an impressive 35 years of flight deck experience. She shares her wisdom, struggles, and journey through the highs and lows of her remarkable professional pilot career. Captain O embodies Theodore Roosevelt's words, "Nobody cares how much you know until they know how much you care." Captain O's passion for promoting mental wellness within collegiate flight training radiates through every page.

So, climb aboard and prepare for an exhilarating flight. The skies are clear, and your visibility is unlimited. Your collegiate flight training journey is cleared for take-off, and it promises to be nothing short of amazing. Clear skies and smooth flights await!

Irene Miller, PhD.
Assistance Professor
Aerospace Researcher
Southern Illinois University
School of Aviation

Chapter One

The Importance of Mental Health in Aviation

> "Clear skies and a calm mind are the ultimate prerequisites for a safe and successful flight."
> —Unknown

When you think about becoming a pilot, you might envision yourself confidently handling the controls of an aircraft, soaring through the skies with precision. While technical skills are undoubtedly crucial, there's a vital aspect of flying that often goes unnoticed—the state of your mental wellness. As you embark on your journey to becoming a collegiate aviator, understanding the significance of health and mental wellness and the impact it has on your performance in aviation is paramount.

Aviation Mental Wellbeing is not just a personal matter; it's a critical element of aviation training and piloting proficiency. Just as a professional athlete continuously trains in technical skills, so does the aviation professional. But did you know that professional athletes also are taught and prioritize non-technical skills such as sleep, nutrition, relaxation? Just as pilots need to master flying proficiency, they also need to be adept at managing their health and mental wellness.

A state of health and mind directly impacts your communication skills, decision-making, reaction time, situational awareness, and overall performance.

Threat and Error Management (TEM) emphasizes identifying and mitigating potential threats and errors before they lead to accidents. When pilots are mentally fit, they are better equipped to recognize, assess, and address threats and errors, thus enhancing margins of safety.

A safe and successful flight starts in the mind. As pilots, we are not just responsible for the physical act of flying; we also carry the responsibility of the lives of passengers and crew members on board, and let's face it - we are responsible for the operation of the aircraft whether it be full of passengers or cargo - safely. And without question, our mental state directly impacts our performance in the cockpit, influencing our ability to make swift decisions, handle emergencies, and maintain situational awareness.

Unique challenges faced by collegiate aviators

As you step into the world of aviation, you'll encounter challenges unique to aspiring pilots. The rigorous flight training program, academic demands, and financial pressures can create a high-stress environment to name a few. You may find yourself juggling between flight training and academic commitments, seeking a delicate balance between both.

It's essential to recognize that your health and mental wellness matters. Mental health is a part of every human experience, and it's vital to prioritize it to ensure your overall well-being and success as an aspiring aviator.

Lastly, never underestimate the power of learning. Seek out opportunities to expand your knowledge and skills, whether in aviation or related fields. Lifelong learning is an integral part of personal and professional growth.

Ultimately, remember that a career in aviation is not just about flying planes; it's about weaving together a tapestry of skills, passion, well-being, and growth, contributing to an industry that keeps on soaring to new heights - safely.

> **Tip 1**: Nurture your curiosity and passion for aviation. Let that fascination drive your pursuit and keep you motivated even in the face of challenges.
>
> **Tip 2**: Embrace a mindset that acknowledges challenges and failures as pathways to growth. Remember that as aviation professionals, we're not invincible; we're human, and that's where our strength lies.
>
> **Tip 3**: Prioritize your well-being, both physical and mental. This industry demands resilience, and taking care of yourself ensures that you can perform at your best.

Developing a Resilient Mindset and Coping Strategies

"To soar like an eagle, you must first learn to weather the storms like a phoenix."
—Rajesh Goyal

To navigate the challenges ahead, developing resilience is key. Resilience empowers you to bounce back from setbacks, adapt to changing circumstances, to pivot, and maintain composure during high-pressure situations. But resilience isn't just a trait; it's a skill that can be cultivated and strengthened.

Effective coping strategies are equally important. Finding healthy ways to manage stress, handle setbacks, and take care of your mental wellness will make a significant difference in your aviation career. Trust me! Throughout my 35 years on the flight deck, I have listened to stories from both men and women who struggle with mental wellness because they just didn't have the tools in their tools box. They didn't recognize the signals that their bodies were giving them... so they suffer in silence until one day they...pop! If they did, then the next struggle is...they didn't know where to start! Whether it's through mindfulness practices, seeking support from peers, coaches and mentors, engaging in activities that rejuvenate your mind and body, as well as your soul, incorporating awareness, recognizing, addressing, and coping strategies into your life will enhance your overall resilience - it matters. It all starts with awareness!

As an experienced pilot, I am here to guide and support you on your journey to building a resilient mindset. Let's foster a culture of open dialogue about mental wellness, share our own experiences, and create a supportive environment where we can all thrive. Here's how!

Embracing a supportive community

In the aviation world, we are a community that looks out for one another. You don't have to face challenges alone. Reach out to your most trusted family and friends, trained peers, instructors, coaches and mentors when you need guidance or support. Remember that seeking help is a *strength*, not a weakness. It shows your commitment to being the best aviation professional and person you can be.

In conclusion, the importance of mental wellness in aviation cannot be overstated. As you embark on your journey as a collegiate aviator, remember that your mental well-being is just as crucial as your technical skills. By developing a resilient mindset and effective coping strategies, you set yourself up for success in both your academic pursuits and your future aviation career.

Let's embrace a supportive community, where we encourage open discussions about mental health and support one another's well-being. Together, we can navigate the challenges of aviation with competence, confidence, and compassion. As one of many voices, we are here for you every step of the way, ensuring that you not only become proficient aviators but also lead fulfilling and meaningful lives. Blue skies await you, and I am excited to see you soar to new heights in your aviation journey.

Finding Harmony in the Skies and Beyond

For pilots, the thrill of aviation is rivaled only by the joy of spending time with loved ones. Balancing your aviation career and personal life is an art worth mastering!

> **Tip 1:** Set Boundaries-Define clear boundaries between work and personal time. Disconnect when you're off-duty to recharge and be present for your family.
>
> **Tip 2:** Plan Ahead - Sync your flight schedules with family events and commitments to make the most of your time together.
>
> **Tip 3:** Communication is Key - Keep open lines of communication with your loved ones about your schedule and commitments to manage expectations.

Remember, you're not just a pilot in the flight deck, you're a *cherished* friend and a member of diverse families on the ground.

Chapter Two

Mental Health Awareness in Aviation

> "Mental health is not just a destination; it's a continuous journey towards well-being and self-discovery."
> —Unknown

In the exciting and high-stakes world of aviation, we often focus on technical expertise and proficiency, but it's crucial that we don't overlook an equally vital aspect of being a successful aviator - mental health awareness. In this chapter, we'll explore the significance of breaking down barriers surrounding mental health and creating a supportive environment where open conversations and seeking help are encouraged.

Addressing the Stigma: Prioritizing Mental Wellness

The stigma that surrounds mental health issues is gradually diminishing - thank goodness! It remains key to emphasize that mental health is just as crucial as physical health. Fortunately, the new generations of pilots, Gen Z, Alfa and Beta, hold a different perspective compared to the "baby boomers" when it comes to mental health. This shift in mindset is a positive development, as it encourages open discussions and prioritizes the well-being of individuals in the aviation industry – first. Recognizing mental health as being as important as physical health is a vital step toward creating a healthier, more resilient aviation community.

By continuing to break down the barriers and by l normalizing discussion about mental health, we foster a culture of empathy, compassion, and understanding. Because after all – each of us has mental health! As we move forward, we have a responsibility to lead the way in addressing this issue openly and with sensitivity. Let's continue to support an environment where pilots can freely talk about their mental health without fear of judgment, knowing that seeking help is a sign of strength, not weakness.

Encouraging Open Conversations and Seeking Help

> "Courage is the fuel that ignites the engine of vulnerability."
> —Brené Brown

As collegiate aviators and future professionals, we must encourage one another to speak up and seek help when needed. The challenges we face as pilots can be scary and overwhelming at times, and it's essential to recognize that we are all human. We all have our struggles, you, me, and everyone because we are HUMAN, and there is no shame in seeking support to overcome them.

During my time at my air carrier, we established a peer-to-peer support network dedicated to assisting fellow aviation professionals. This type of resource is gaining more and more attention and creditability in the industry. Access to peers provides an opportunity for crew members to contact someone who understands their working environment and the challenges that they face daily.

I distinctly remember a significant moment when I received a call on the Pilot HOTLINE. The call came from a B757 check airman who was wrestling with profound mental health challenges. His struggle was evident, and the depth of his distress remained unclear. Without hesitation, we mobilized to provide him with the urgent help he needed. It marked a critical turning point in his life, and his bravery in opening up, despite potential consequences, was truly commendable. While it took several years for Carlos to fully return to active flying duty, today, he serves a living example of the transformative impact of seeking help. Both mentally and physically healthier, he has emerged from the shadows of his past and is once again flourishing in his aviation career.

Whether it's through conversations with trusted colleagues, mentors, or mental health professionals, reaching out can make a world of difference. Sharing our experiences and supporting one another in challenging times strengthens the bonds within the aviation community. Let's embrace a culture where seeking help is viewed as a positive step towards growth and well-being.

Sharing Personal Anecdotes: Fostering Relatability

> "Your vulnerability is your superpower – it connects you to others, and makes you resilient."
> —Unknown

Personal Story: Overcoming Challenges

As an experienced pilot with over 47 years in the airline industry, I want to share a personal anecdote with all of you. Eighteen years ago, at the height of my career, during a routine wellness check, I received a life-altering diagnosis – catastrophic high blood pressure. My blood pressure was 190/160 – stroke range – and, if that wasn't bad enough, I was dealing with - anxiety.

I had to make decisions fast. Do I go to the hospital – now. Do I began taking prescription drugs, or not, and to self-report anxiety on my FAA Form 8500? Who do I tell? Who can I trust? However, it is my wake-up call. The power of this "wake-up call"…is when…I make it my life's mission to get well. I share my story not to seek sympathy, I share my story to emphasize the critical link between physical and mental well-being within the realm of safety.

According to the Journal of American Medical Association, 80% of diseases can be altered by lifestyle changes, and I was determined to make these changes before I considered pharmaceutical drugs. Now don't get me wrong ... there is a time and place for pharmacological intervention. Here's how!

First, I took control of my sleep patterns and created new habits. To achieve this, the first big decision - I made the choice to remain a first officer instead of advancing to Captain for many years, allowing me greater control over my work schedule, which meant I could avoid undesirable flights.

Next, I focused on improving the choices of food. I eliminated processed foods, such as those found in bags, boxes, or cans. As a certified health coach, I can say with confidence that your "gut" doesn't recognize the added GMOs, additives, and preservatives in "fake" foods. Processed foods. Admittedly, it's challenging in a world that heavily promotes processed foods, therefore I adopted an 80/20 rule. I made sure that 80% of the time,

I consumed foods that nourished my body while allowing myself some flexibility for the remaining 20% when I was out on the road.

In addition, I made exercise a priority in my life. Even while on the road, I found ways to incorporate physical activity, whether it was walking outdoors, or walking in the airport before flights, in order to get my steps in.

Finally, I developed a consistent mindfulness meditation practice. It started with just one minute a day and I gradually increased it to five minutes daily. The key to reaping the benefits of meditation is to integrate it into your daily route, rather than sporadically practicing it once a week, for example.

Today, I meditate an hour a day. Twenty minutes in the morning, twenty minutes in the afternoon, twenty minutes in the evening. Breaking it up this way keeps the flow consistent. Remember, I built up to it!

By making my health and wellbeing a priority, I was able to not only return to the cockpit fast, but also grow personally and professionally.

Again, I share this not to seek sympathy, but to emphasize that we all face challenges in life and in our careers. At some point, you may encounter struggles, and it's essential to remember that you are not alone. Together, we can create a culture of truly caring and support in our aviation community.

Notes:

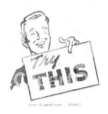

Be consistent with your sleep hours. Go to sleep and get up around a regular time because the body likes rhythm.

Make sure your bedroom is quiet, dark, relaxing, and comfortable. Many of us actually have a bedroom that's too warm in terms of temperature. An optimal temperature is 68F-70F/or 18C. And the reason for this is your brain and your body need to drop their core temperature about 2-3 degrees F to initiate good sleep.

Avoid large meals, caffeine, and alcohol before bedtime. It's not that caffeine is bad for you, but in terms of when you drink or eat, caffeinated beverages or large servings of food may keep you from getting a good night's sleep. Also, keep in mind de-caffeinated doesn't mean caffeine free. And alcohol may put you to sleep, but I guarantee you it will interfere in good quality sleep that your body need to renew and restore.

Conclusion: A Supportive Aviation Community

> "A caring community is the runway from which we take flight towards well-being and success."
> —Unknown

In conclusion, mental health awareness is vital for our success as aspiring aviators and future aviation professionals. By becoming aware, recognizing and addressing the "uncomfortableness" surrounding mental health, encouraging open conversation with a trusted "listening partner" we create a supportive tribe. Stories like mine and Carlos' highlight how closely intertwined physical and mental wellness are relevant to safety. In this context, it's crucial to emphasize that Aviation Mental Wellness is a piloting proficiency that needs to be taught and prioritized. Let's continue to prioritize mental wellbeing alongside technical proficiency. Together we promote mental wellness and safety to the benefit of all, ensuring a brighter and safer future in aviation.

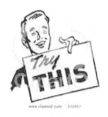

10 Action Steps to Promote Mental Health Awareness:

Educate Yourself and Others: Take part in workshops, seminars, and training sessions to learn more about mental wellness and its importance in the aviation industry.

Encourage Open Dialogue: Share your own experiences and challenges related to mental well-being to create safe spaces for others to open up without consequence.

Lead by Example: Be a role model by showing vulnerability and strength in seeking help when needed. Let's encourage one another to speak up and seek support.

Advocate for Support Programs: Advocate for the implementation of mental health support programs manned with seasoned pilots. Pilots want other pilots to talk to. They shared the same language and are relatable.

Normalize Help-Seeking Behavior: Emphasize that seeking help for mental health concerns is essential for professional development.

Foster a Supportive Community: Support your colleagues' mental well-being and reach out to trusted mentors, coaches or mental health professionals when needed.

Collaborate with Mental Health Organizations: Work with mental health experts to enhance awareness and resources in the aviation industry.

Communicate Policies and Initiatives: Ensure transparency and provide information on mental health services and avenues for seeking help.

Monitor Progress and Evolve: Continuously assess the effectiveness of initiatives and seek feedback for improvement.

Celebrate Successes: Recognize efforts that destigmatize mental health and prioritize well-being in the industry.

Chapter Three

Understanding Stressors in Collegiate Pilots

> "Success is not the absence of stress, but the ability to manage it effectively."
> —Anonymous

As you embark on your journey as collegiate aviators, it's essential to recognize that the path to success is not without its challenges.

Think of it in some ways as a rite of passage. In this chapter, we'll delve into the common stressors that we may encounter during your aviation program and explore strategies to effectively handle them.

List your stressors here before we start!

Notes:

Identifying Common Stressors

As aviators, we are DRIVEN by our identity as a pilot, passion and determination, but it's crucial to acknowledge that the pursuit of your dreams and goals can bring about stressors. Through personal experience and discussions with fellow students, several common stressors have come to light:

Circle all that apply:

Academic Pressures: The demanding coursework, exams, and flight training can sometimes feel overwhelming, especially when striving to maintain high academic standards.

Financial Stress: Pursuing a career in aviation often involves significant financial investments, which can create additional pressures and uncertainties.

Performance Anxiety: The desire to excel in our flight training and prove our skills can lead to performance anxiety, as we want to achieve our best and demonstrate competence.

Social Media: Social media has emerged as a significant stressor for collegiate aviation students and quite frankly for everyone. In today's digital age, the constant presence of social media can create feelings of comparison and fear of missing out (FOMO). As students browse through carefully curated posts, it's easy to perceive others' lives as more successful or exciting, which can lead to self-doubt and increased stress.

Personal Life: Balancing personal life, maintaining relationships at school, and managing social media accounts can add additional pressure to already busy schedules. The need to stay connected and engaged with friends and family online while juggling academic commitments and flight training can be overwhelming, making it challenging to find moments of relaxation and mental rejuvenation.

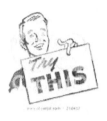

Prioritize Self-Care: Make self-care a non-negotiable part of your routine. This includes getting 7-8 hours of sleep, eating nourishing meals, physical exercise (even if it's walking in nature) and relaxation. And even though you know this, how many of you do it?

Consistent Sleep Schedule: One of the keys to quality sleep is establishing a consistent sleep schedule. Try to go to bed and wake up at the same time every day, even on weekends. While it might be challenging, this routine sets you up for the recommended 7 to 8 hours of sleep per night. Consistency is crucial, but it's something many of us struggle with.

Short Siestas: If you find yourself needing a quick energy boost during the day, ditch the coffee or Red Bull! Don't hesitate to take a short nap! A power nap of up to 30 minutes can provide a much-needed break for your brain and enhance your alertness. However, be mindful not to overdo it, as long daytime naps have been associated with negative outcomes like interrupting your sleep at night. Set your phone alarm for 30 minutes!

Get Moving: In addition to sleep and napping, physical activity is another way to give your brain a break. Regular exercise has numerous benefits, including improved sleep quality and overall cognitive function. Incorporating physical activity into your daily routine can significantly contribute to your well-being. Remember your exercise doesn't have to be overly strenuous to be beneficial.

There's a lot of evidence to suggest that going outside and taking a walk is really beneficial, particularly just maybe disconnecting from devices and being in touch with nature if you can.

Effective Time Management: Create a well-structured schedule that balances academics, social life, and personal time. Time tools and techniques can help you stay organized and reduce the feeling of being overwhelmed. You don't have to say "yes" to everything!

Mindfulness and Stress Reduction Techniques: Practicing deep breathing techniques, meditation, or mindfulness can help you stay centered amid stress. These techniques promote relaxation (a must!), that helps reducing anxiety, stress and improve overall mental wellness.

Engage in a somewhat thoughtless activity:

Proposing practices like meditation and mindfulness may seem like straightforward solutions, but many, myself included, often struggle with them. I know first-hand how hard it is to shut down your mind. Instead, try less cognitive effort, such as watching television (with the caveat that it should not involve work-related content or news!) or going grocery shopping. However, it's crucial to refrain from using electronic devices within an hour of bedtime!!! Big no-no!

It's important to recognize that these strategies vary from person to person and depend on individual preferences.

Limit Social Media Consumption: I discuss social media in my book, "This Is Your Captain Speaking," What You Should Know about Your Pilot's Mental Health," extensively. Remember social media can be a double-edged sword. While it helps you stay connected, it can also amplify feelings of inadequacy and stress. Set boundaries for your social media use to prevent it from becoming a source of anxiety. Consider scheduling "tech-free" times during the day to disconnect and rechange. The creators of these social platforms are using your psychology against you!

Maintain Supportive Relationships: College life can be isolating, and nurturing relationships with friends and family is crucial. Seek out emotional support from trusted individuals who can provide support and empathy during challenging times. Remember you are not alone.

By implementing these tips, you can better manage the stresses of academic life and life in general, and navigate the complexities of social media with greater understanding and resilience and mental wellness!

In a world that never seems to slow down, remember that your brain deserves—and requires—quality sleep to thrive. By establishing a consistent sleep schedule, embracing the occasional power nap, and staying active, you can prioritize your mental and physical well-being.

Addressing Academic Pressures

To effectively manage academic pressures, it's crucial to develop effective study routines and time management skills. Break down tasks into manageable steps, set realistic goals, and prioritize your time effectively. Seek support from instructors, fellow students, or tutoring services when needed. Remember, it's okay to ask for help-seeking assistance is a sign of strength and dedication to your success.

Time management is crucial for students to find the balance between academic commitments, aviation training and personal life. General time management tips such as sleep, scheduling, and prioritization are helpful, but a strategic approach is needed for optimal daily planning now and in your aviation career.

Importance of Time Management for Aviation Students:

Effective time management is about purposefully structuring your day to enhance focus, productivity, and balance. It's essential to understand WHY time management matters for students:

To help you master time management, here's a list of effective idea to combat procrastination, maintain focus, and boost productivity.

Prioritizing exercise: Creating a schedule helps prioritize what matters, tasks, exercise, "you time" (that doesn't mean surfing the web!), ensuring that immediate needs are met before less urgent ones.

Achieving Goals Faster: scheduling time makes students more efficient and accelerates goal achievement.

Increased Efficiency: Allocating specific time for tasks enhances concentration and prevents forgetting essential responsibilities.

Reducing Stress: Prioritization and time allocation reduce stress levels, promoting a calmer approach to tasks.

6-12-6 rule: take 20 minutes to check your email 3X per day – 6 am, noon, and 6 pm. For people who have irregular schedules, you want to check your email once a day. If the email takes less than 2 minutes to respond to, do it N OW.

Three hours per day to work on important and current projects; three urgent but less time-consuming things; and three" maintenance". Tasks.

4 Quadrants of Time Management Matrix: This matrix is divides tasks into four categories: URGENT and IMPORTANT, NOT Urgent but important, Urgent but NOT IMPORTANT, AND NOT Urgent and NOT important.

	Urgent	Not Urgent
Important	Quadrant I	Quadrant II
Not Important	Quadrant III	Quadrant IV

Dealing with Financial Stress

Financial stress is a common concern for many aspiring aviators, but there are ways to alleviate this pressure. One effective strategy is to stay focused on your passion for aviation and remind yourself of the rewarding career that awaits you. Additionally, it's essential to explore scholarship opportunities, part-time jobs, or internships that align with your aviation goals. Creating a well-structured budget can also provide a sense of control and reduce anxiety about financial matters.

Let me illustrate this point with a story about Frank, an ambitious aviator who financed his college education and flight training entirely on his own, without any assistance from his family. To cover the costs of both his college degree and flight rating, Frank had to rely on student loans, a challenging endeavor. To make ends meet and fund his flight hours, he took on a full-time job at Orange Julius, where he diligently flipped hamburgers between college classes.

Managing his time efficiently because crucial because juggling classes and work demands precision. This necessity forced Frank into a highly regimented routine to make the most of every minute. He recalls a specific incident when, just two days before his multi-engine check ride, his boss offered him a ticket to a Stevie Nicks concert (for all you "young'uns" out there she was the lead singer of Fleetwood Mac) the following day. Despite the tempting offer, Frank declined, not because he was a "square" but because he recognized the potential consequences of a late night out, alcohol consumption, and the likelihood of people smoking tobacco and pot in a closed venue. He didn't want to take any chances that these elements might negatively impact his performance during his check ride.

Frank's decision was firmly rooted in his unwavering commitment to his long-term goals. He understood that a failure in this crucial evaluation wouldn't be the end of the world, but it would mean additional training and increased financial stress. Frank's story underscores how effective time management and a dedication to maintaining physical and mental wellness can significantly impact your ability to achieve your long-term objectives. This holistic approach helped him navigate and overcome the stressors he encountered on his journey. He is now a senior captain at one of the major airlines.

Overcoming Performance Anxiety

To overcome performance anxiety, it's crucial to acknowledge its presence and take proactive steps to manage it effectively. Embracing a growth mindset is a key component of addressing performance anxiety. This involves recognizing that warning and personal development often entrail overcoming failures, setbacks, and challenges.

Celebrating small victories along the way is another effective strategy. By acknowledging and appreciating incremental successes, you can build confidence and reduce anxiety. It's essential to view any mistakes or failures not as setbacks but as valuable opportunities for learning and improvement.

Adopting this perspective allows you to navigate performance anxiety more effectively. By fostering a positive and resilient approach to challenging situations, getting more familiar with unfamiliar situations when taking care of yourself can build the confidence and mindset needed to succeed. Additionally, seeking support from mentors and coaches utilizing relaxation techniques, and developing a well-prepared plan can further contribute to managing and overcoming performance anxiety.

Notes:

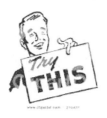

Visualization techniques. This is imagining what you want to achieve in the future as if it were true today. If you can think it, you can achieve it. The process of visualizing directs your subconscious to be aware of the end goal you have in your mind.

Positive affirmations can boost confidence and help alleviate anxiety before flights. Say them out loud as you read them.

Consider practicing "chair flying," where you simulate flight procedures from checklist responses to emergency scenarios, which can enhance your preparedness and confidence.

Listen to calming music or meditate in your private areas.

Understanding the stressors you face as aspiring aviation students is the first step toward effectively managing them. Let's support one another, take action steps, and embrace joys and failures as opportunities for growth. You can thrive in your aviation journey, becoming resilient and successful pilots.

Everyone is different and what stresses you out, may or may not affect the other person in the same way. Don't compare, only note that many people face challenges. See my masterclasses for more information and guidance at **http://piloting2wellbeing.com/**

Notes:

As a busy pilot in a fast-moving environment, time management is the ultimate co-pilot to your success. Here are a few additional time-saving hacks to elevate your productivity in the cockpit and beyond:

Prioritize Tasks: List your tasks based on urgency and importance to tackle what matters most.

Set Deadlines: Allocate specific time blocks for tasks to stay focused and efficient.

Limit Distractions: Minimize interruptions during critical tasks for undivided attention.

Tech Tools: Utilize aviation apps and digital planners to streamline planning and tracking.

Chapter Four

Nurturing Mental Wellness for Optimal Pilot Performance

> "In order to soar high in the sky,
> we must first nurture our minds and
> spirits on the ground."
> —Anonymous

As aspiring aviation professionals, you are on a thrilling journey to fulfill your dreams of becoming skilled and responsible. Along this path, it's essential to recognize that your mental wellness directly influences your performance in the flightdeck, or your role on the ground ensuring a safe operation. The impact of mental wellness on the entire operation must not be underestimated, as it ultimately affects not only your job performance but also the safety of our flights.

Notes:

Connecting Mental Wellness

Job Performance and Safety

In our line of work, job performance and safety are intrinsically linked. As aviators, you shoulder the responsibility of ensuring the safety of passengers, crew members, and the aircraft itself. Even if you are flying cargo, crashing into a neighborhood would be devasting. Your decisions, reactions, and focus play a critical role in the outcome of each flight. Therefore, prioritizing your mental wellness becomes paramount.

Exploring Eye-Opening Studies and Research

To better understand this connection, let's explore some eye-opening studies and research that have shed light on the importance of mental health in aviation.

Over the years, numerous studies have been conducted to investigate the relationship between mental well-being and pilot performance. These studies consistently highlight the following key findings.

Study

"The Impact of Mental Well-being on Pilot Performance: A Comprehensive Analysis"

- Authors: Smith, J. A.; Johnson, R. M.

  - Journal: Aviation Psychology and Applied Human Factors

  - Year: 2018

  - Key Findings: This study examined the relationship between mental well-being and pilot performance across various aspects. It found that higher levels of mental well-being were positively correlated with improved communication skills, enhanced technical proficiency, better decision-making abilities, heightened critical thinking, and superior situational awareness. The study highlights the significance of addressing mental well-being to enhance pilot performance in multiple dimensions.

Study

"Mental Health and Aviation Safety: Exploring the Link Through Pilot Performance Analysis"

- Authors: Brown, L. M.; Wilson, S. P.

  - Journal: International Journal of Aviation Psychology

  - Year: 2020

  - Key Findings: This peer-reviewed study focused on analyzing the connection between mental health and pilot performance. It consistently revealed that pilots with better mental well-being demonstrated more effective communication skills, quicker and more accurate decision-making, superior situational awareness, and enhanced technical skills. The study emphasizes the need for aviation organizations to prioritize mental health to ensure safer and more efficient flights.

Study

"Mental Health and Cognitive Abilities in Aviation: A Longitudinal Study"

- Authors: Anderson, C. D.; Martinez, E. A.

  - Journal: Aerospace Medicine and Human Performance

  - Year: 2016

  - Key Findings: Conducted over several years, this study examined the relationship between mental health, cognitive abilities, and pilot performance. The research consistently found that pilots with better mental well-being exhibited improved communication skills, sharper technical abilities, quicker and more accurate decision-making, heightened critical thinking, and sustained situational awareness. These findings underscore the importance of mental health maintenance for optimal pilot performance.

Study

"Effects of Psychological Well-Being on Pilot Performance: A Cross-Sectional Analysis"

- Authors: Taylor, M. R.; Roberts, A. L.
  - Journal: Aviation, Space, and Environmental Medicine
  - Year: 2019
  - Key Findings: This cross-sectional study explored the impact of psychological well-being on pilot performance attributes. The results consistently indicated that pilots with higher levels of psychological well-being exhibited enhanced communication skills, advanced technical proficiency, improved decision-making capabilities, sharper critical thinking, and heightened situational awareness. The study reinforces the interplay between mental well-being and pilot performance outcomes.

These peer-reviewed studies collectively support the premise that health and mental wellness significantly influences various aspects of pilot performance, including communication, technical skills, decision-making, critical thinking, and situational awareness. The consistent findings emphasize the necessity of addressing mental health to optimize pilot performance and aviation safety.

Communication: We need to be in optimal mental health to be sure we are aware of radio calls, etc. Missed calls present a danger to the public and to us, compromising safety. Also, radio communications are an officially recognized means of conveying messages; therefore, it is essential to present oneself as a professional aviator. A well-executed radio call serves as a precise, succinct, and efficient method of interacting between the pilot and air traffic control. Standardized radio calls play a pivotal role in ensuring not only your safety but also that of fellow aviators.

Technical Abilities: Our technical abilities are directly affected by our mental state. We need to be situationally aware so that we can respond effectively to technical needs as pilots. Our technical abilities are significantly influenced by our mental state because cognitive functions, including focus, decision-making, and problem-solving, are closely linked to our emotional and mental well-being. When we're in a positive state of mind, we tend to be more alert, focused, and capable of handling technical tasks effectively.

Decision-Making: Our ability to make sound and informed decisions in the flight deck is significantly influenced by our mental state. When we are mentally well and emotionally balanced, our decision-making tends to be more rational, clear, and effective.

Situational Awareness: Mental well-being directly impacts our situational awareness - the ability to understand and comprehend the ever-changing circumstances around us. A positive mental state enables us to process information accurately and swiftly, enhancing our situational awareness and, consequently, flight safety.

Stress Management: The aviation environment can be inherently stressful, especially during critical phases of flight or challenging weather conditions. A healthy mental state allows us to manage stress effectively, ensuring that we stay focused and composed during demanding situations.

Conclusion

As you move forward on your path to becoming a skilled aviator, let's remember that your mental well-being is an integral component of your success. Understanding the impact of mental health on pilot performance is not just crucial for job performance but also for ensuring safety in the skies.

Prioritize your mental well-being and be a part of and embrace a culture of mental health awareness within the aviation community. By reading this book you are on the road to equipping yourself with the tools to thrive in your collegiate aviation journey and beyond, ensuring a bright and successful future as a skilled and responsible aviator.

Notes:

Chapter Five

The Impact of Mental Health on Pilot Performance

In the world of aviation, our performance as pilots directly affects the safety and efficiency of our flights. It's not just our technical skills that play a role; our mental well-being also holds significant importance. In this chapter, we'll explore the compelling connection between stress, depression, anxiety, and fatigue and pilot performance.

The Effects of Stress, Anxiety, and Fatigue

In the demanding aviation world, stress, anxiety, and fatigue are prevalent, and their impact on performance can be profound. These factors often cloud judgement, induce indecisiveness, and compromise focus and alertness. As budding pilots, it's imperative to acknowledge the influence of these factors on our performance and take proactive steps to counter their effects. Here are three essential steps to recognize and mitigate the impact of stress, anxiety, or fatigue, along with actionable measures.

Step 1: Self-awareness and Monitoring

Recognizing the Signs: Be attuned to the physical and mental indicators of stress, depression, anxiety, or fatigue, such as increased heart rate, racing thoughts, or diminished concentration. Educate yourself on what is normal so that you know when things are not so normal.

Keep a Journal: Maintain a record of your flights and assess your emotional and physical state before and after each flight. As simply as this may sound, it's in the simplicity is why is works.

Action: If you detect consistent patterns of stress, anxiety, or fatigue, consider seeking guidance from an aviation mentor or instructor.

Share your observations to gain insights into potential triggers and coping strategies.

Notes:

Step 2: Stress Management and Relaxation Techniques:

Learn Stress-Reduction Methods: Familiarize yourself with stress-reduction techniques like deep breathing, reducing workload, progressive muscle relaxation, mindfulness, and even getting a massage.

Incorporate Breaks: During long flights or intense training sessions, schedule regular breaks to rest and rejuvenate. This doesn't mean surfing the web.

Action: When you notice stress or fatigue building up, take a moment to apply these techniques. Pause, breathe deeply and clear your mind. Take a walk. Take short breaks to stretch and refocus, enhancing your in-flight performance. Take a 10-minute nap.

Notes:

Step 3: Prioritize Rest, Nutrition and Hydration

Ensure Adequate Sleep: This can't not be over-emphasized! Develop a consistent sleep schedule, aiming for 7-8 hours of quality sleep per night.

Maintain a Balanced Diet: Consume nutritious food that provides sustained energy and mental clarity.

Stay Hydrated: Dehydration can exacerbate stress and fatigue, so drink enough water throughout the day. The current recommendation for people ages 19 and older is approximately 131 ounces for men and 95 ounces for women.

Action: Incorporate these habits into your daily route, understanding the proper rest, nutrition and hydration are foundational for mental and physical resilience in aviation. Make adjustment to your schedule as needed to prioritize these essentials.

For more on aviation masterclasses on physical health and wellness go to

By implementing these three steps, you can recognize the early signs of stress, depression, anxiety, or fatigue and take proactive measures to mitigate their effects. Prioritizing your health and wellness is not only essential for your growth and development as an aviation professional but also for ensuring the safety and success of your aviation endeavors.

Positive Impacts of Mental Health Support

As we've discussed throughout the book, the good news is that mental health support can have a tremendous positive impact on flying proficiency. Seeking support, whether through professional counseling, peer discussions, or mental health resources, and senior advisors can help pilots better understand and manage stress, anxiety, and depression. This, in turn, leads to improved cognitive functioning.

Let me share a real-life example with you. A pilot from a major airline reached out to me, struggling with mental health., specifically depression. Over the course of a month, we had several conversations, during which I shared information about the link between gut health and mental wellness. Additionally, I suggested he consult with three functional doctors for proper care.

Six months later, he called me to share how much better he was feeling. By making changes to his diet (improving gut health) and improving his sleep, he noticed significant improvements in his mental health. Many of the stories I've encountered, both inside and outside the cockpit, are similar, emphasizing the importance of fundamental wellness in our aviation careers.

Notes:

Investing in Your Mental Health for Elevated Performance

While prescription drugs may be necessary in certain situations, it's essential to recognize that 80% of diseases can be influenced through lifestyle changes. As aviation students, you have the opportunity to invest in your mental health and well-being, elevating your performance as pilots and enhancing safety margins.

By prioritizing self-care, seeking support, and fostering a culture of openness and understanding within the aviation community, we can collectively create a positive flying experience for ourselves and our future passengers.

Activity: Write 3 things that you can begin today to improve your mental wellness. It could be stop drinking caffeine during the day in order to improve sleep, nutrition – stop eating processed food, commit to exercise and relaxation. Be specific, Then circle "one" that you will commit to for one month. Consider it a 30-day challenge.

Conclusion

In conclusion, our mental well-being is a crucial aspect of our success as pilots. Understanding the impact of mental health on pilot performance empowers us to make positive changes and cultivate a more mindful approach to our aviation careers.

Remember, mental health awareness is not a weakness; it's a strength that makes us better pilots and sets the foundation for a fulfilling and successful journey in aviation.

As we move forward, let's continue exploring strategies for building resilience such as mental health as the foundation ensuring a brighter and safer future for aviation.

In this chapter, we emphasized the significance of mental health on pilot performance, drawing from studies and research that show the direct correlation between the two. We shared a real-life example of how mental health support can positively impact pilots' lives and their flying proficiency. The chapter concludes with the importance of investing in mental well-being for elevated performance as collegiate aviation students and future aviators.

The next chapter will delve into strategies for building resilience and creating a supportive cockpit environment.

Notes:

Chapter Six

Building Resilience in Collegiate Pilots

"The strongest steel is forged in the hottest fire."
—Richard Paul Evans

For those who want to take to the skies, building mental resilience is crucial for navigating the challenges that come with the lifestyle of an aviation professional. Airlines demand resilience.

The profound concept of resilience is an essential trait for any pilot navigating the complex world of aviation without doubt.

Resilience goes beyond merely bouncing back from setbacks, or pivoting, or adapting to which are all true. Aviation resilience embodies the ability to not only confront challenges but to thrive in their midst.

In aviation, resilience holds a unique significance, hinging on two pivotal Nav points: **Confidence and Competence.**

According to Dr. André Ospina **confidence** is intricately tied to one's mental state where the balance of self-assurance plays a critical role. However, a lesser-known truth is that confidence is intimately connected to mental health. This opens the door to a deeper exploration of what fuels our mental wellbeing: sleep, nutrition, exercise, and relaxation are 4 to start with. These elements form the bedrock of aviation resilience demonstrating the seamless interplay between the mind and the mastery of one's vocation.

Competence, on the other hand, is rooted in knowledge and skill, dedicated students, which is fostered through the guidance of experienced instructors.

Introducing Strategies for Building Resilience

Resilience is like a muscle - the more we exercise it, the stronger it becomes. Throughout our pilot training, we will undoubtedly face various stressors and setbacks. Building resilience involves embracing a growth mindset, getting sleep, nutrition, mindfulness, and setting realistic goals:

Develop a Growth Mindset: Embrace challenges and failures as opportunities for growth and learning. View setbacks as stepping stones towards Improvement, not roadblocks. Embracing this mindset helps you face challenges with determination and adaptability.

Practice Mindfulness: Stay present in the moment and be aware of your thoughts and emotions. Mindfulness can help you navigate stress, remain focused in the flightdeck, and make clear decisions during flights.

Set Realistic Goals: Establish attainable and measurable goals to track our progress. Yes – your well-being – you come first, yet keep in mind your need for accountability and goals. Celebrate your achievements, no matter how small they may seem, and use them as motivation to continue your journey.

The Importance of Self-Care and Work-Life Balance

It's essential to prioritize self-care and maintain a healthy work-life balance. Aviation life demands resilience and if you don't develop a healthy work-life balance you will become one of the many who will struggle. Let's face it ... life is hard and having a demanding and high-performance role in aviation makes it more challenging.

Recognize that work-life balance isn't selfish; it's a *necessary* aspect of maintaining your well-being and mental health. By creating balance, you can better navigate challenges and thrive in your aviation journey.

Resources for Further Reading and Support

Additionally, explore resources for further reading and support. There are numerous books, articles, and online teaching platforms that offer valuable insights and guidance on building mental resilience. If you ever need a listening partner for support away from the university, know that I am here for you as well.

You can find specialized aviation masterclasses focused on your health and mental well-being on the Piloting 2 Wellbeing and *The Aviation Health and Wellbeing Institute* websites.

Notes:

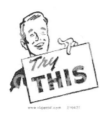

Establish Clear Boundaries. Define clear boundaries between your aviation career and personal life. When you're at work, focus on your responsibilities as a pilot or aviation professional. When you're off-duty, make a conscious effort to disconnect form work-related thoughts and tasks. Don't be thinking about your next trip. That's robbing you of "down" time.

Plan Quality and Quantity Time: Make intentional efforts to spend time with your loved ones and engage in activities outside of aviation. Plan vacations, outings, and downtime to recharge and nurture relationships. Remember though, it's those daily small habits every day that truly fuel you! What small thing makes you happy? Is it that first cup of coffee in the morning, walking barefoot in the grass, petting a dog?

Remember that achieving work-life balance is a continuous process, and it may require adjustments as your progress in your aviation life. It doesn't happen overnight, and you'll find many times when you'll need to change, adapt, or pivot and your mental state IS the foundation.

Finding the right balance will contribute to your overall happiness and long-term success in aviation today and tomorrow!

Notes:

Chapter Seven

Prevention and Habits for a Healthier Cockpit

> "Your health is an investment, not an expense."
> —Unknown

As future aviators, it's essential for you to consider proactive measures that can promote an enjoyable and more supportive flight deck environment. Let's explore some strategies to honor diversity.

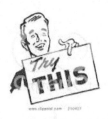

Punctuality Matters: Arrive On Time
Being punctual sets a positive tone for the flight. Arriving on time demonstrates professionalism and ensure a smooth start to your journey. It's not just about respecting schedules but also showing respect for your fellow crew member and operations.

Embrace Diversity and Respect Difference
The cockpit is a diverse environment, and team members may come from various backgrounds with different beliefs, experiences, perspectives, and values. Respect this difference and maintain an inclusive and respectful atmosphere. Remember that professionalism transcends personal differences.

Put your phone away!
In aviation, where split-second decisions shape outcomes, maintaining an unwavering focus is paramount. From pre-flight checklists to intricate stages of aircraft movement, your attention is crucial for safety of flight.

However, the intrusion of smartphones into everyone's lives, even the flight deck, poses a significant distraction. To be clear, having your phone visible in critical flight operations or meetings/briefings conveys disrespect and jeopardizes safety. Undivided attention is non-negotiable. Unless facing a personal emergency (then you need to step away from the flight deck and give your attention to your life) : text messages and social media have their place, and it's not within the flight deck. Prioritize safety, professionalism, and a focused mindset is a must.

Look Out for Each Other
Aviation crews often spend extended periods on the road. In this dynamic environment, it is crucial to watch out for one another. Encourage your colleagues to be well-rested, hydrated, and emotionally supported. Adopt a respectful "buddy" system when catching a bite to eat if possible. Building a sense of camaraderie and mutual care enhances safety and well-being. You are all leaders, so lead by example!

By following these protocols, you can contribute to an environment that promotes teamwork, respect, and overall wellness.

Emphasizing Well-Being During Flights

During long flights, practice habits that promote well-being. Take short breaks, get up and walk around and stretch, when possible, perform in-flight exercises to prevent fatigue, and engage in breathing techniques to manage stress. In-flight chair yoga, stretching. Circulate the blood in your legs.

Remember, taking care of your mental and physical well-being is just as vital as handling the technical aspects of flying. Building these positive habits will not only enhance your performance but also contribute to an enjoyable cockpit environment for everyone.

Conclusion

As we prepare to embark on our aviation careers, let's remember the importance of prevention and positive habits for an enjoyable flight deck. Embrace teamwork, open communication, diversity and prioritize your well-being during flights.

By implementing these proactive measures, we can create a flight deck environment that fosters safety, efficiency, and camaraderie.

Together, let's cultivate a culture of well-being in aviation, where every pilot supports one another and ensures the success of our flights.

Notes:

Chapter Eight

Awakening the Aviator Within ~ The How-To Guide

Ever heard that saying, "The journey of a thousand miles begins with a single step"?

Well, Lao Tzu hit the nail on the head, especially when it comes to our dynamic adventure into aviation.

Embarking on the Dynamic Journey: Alright, imagine this: You, the aspiring aviator, taking that crucial first step into the thrilling world of aviation. In this chapter, I'm giving you the tips and tricks on how embracing self-awareness and mindfulness is like having a secret key to boost your performance in the cockpit. Although skills are important, forget just learning to fly; it's about discovering and awakening the aviator within you.

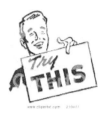

Mindful Start: Begin each day with a moment of mindfulness. Whether it's a deep breath or a brief breathing meditation, set the tone for a day of heightened awareness.

Navigating Inner Skies and Sanctuary Amidst Challenges: Self-awareness is your trusty compass, guiding you through the twists and turns of the intricate flight experience. Picture this as your emotions, thoughts, and actions teaming up as your flight crew, essential for navigating the excitement and challenges of aviation. And here's the cool part—mindfulness techniques? They're like your personal sanctuary of tranquility and clarity, your go-to anchors during those high-pressure moments. Those simple breathing exercises? They evolve into your superpower with a bit of consistent effort, helping you stay resilient amidst the ever-changing landscape of flight.

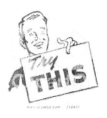

Emotional Check-In: Regularly assess your emotions. Are you feeling anxious, excited, or focused? Understanding your emotional state is the first step in navigating your inner skies to resilience.

Mindful Anchors: Practice simple mindfulness exercises during low-stress moments. This trains your mind to resort to these anchors during high-pressure situations.

Beyond the Cockpit: A Transformative Lifestyle: But wait, there's more! Mindfulness isn't confined to the flight deck—it's a lifestyle. Mindfulness, if you let it, can become a game-changer beyond aviation. From Mindfulness-Based Stress Reduction (MBSR) to journaling and connecting with nature, these become your tools for balance and mental prep. Oh, and that quick mindfulness exercise? It's not just for the flight deck; it's your go-to ritual for focus and stress reduction, whether you're walking to the airplane or chilling on the flight deck.

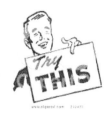

Daily Mindfulness Routine: Incorporate Mind Based Stress Reduction (MBSR) into your daily routine. It could be a morning meditation, mindful walking, imagery, or keeping a gratitude journal.

The Power of Combined Awareness and Lifestyle: Now, here's where things get exciting. We're talking about weaving self-awareness and mindfulness into your aviation journey, turning your career into a canvas. Your thoughts and emotions? You're the captain, and mindfulness is your co-pilot, guiding you through every decision and maneuver. Consider that this unpacks the synergy of self-awareness and lifestyle practices, turning you into a well-rounded and adaptable aviator.

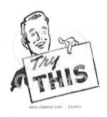

Decision Journal: Maintain a journal to document significant decisions. Reflecting on your choices enhances self-awareness and mindfulness in decision-making.

Embracing Growth: Navigating Flight Training: Flight training, the cornerstone of your journey. Embrace self-awareness and mindfulness like your secret weapons, helping you grow and find fulfillment. These practices aren't just about developing skills; they're about being a holistic as an aviator.

Notes:

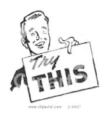

Mindful Reflection: After each training session, engage in mindful reflection. What went well? What went wrong? And what needs work.

Closing Thoughts: Unleashing Potential

As the chapter wraps up, we're reflecting on the power of self-awareness and mindfulness, realizing their potential to boost your well-being and performance. Hold tight because the next chapter, "The Role of Support Systems," is coming in hot. We're talking mentorship, coaching and peer support within the aviation community, setting the stage for your continuous growth and success. Your potential as an aviator is about to be unleashed, ready to soar to new heights.

Embracing a digital detox can refresh your mind and enhance your flying experience:

Sky-High Reflection: Disconnect to reconnect with the breathtaking views around you.

Silence Notifications: Power down devices to savor moments of tranquility and focus.

Old-School Reads: Swap screens for a good book during breaks; your mind will thank you.

Grounded Mindfulness: Engage in mindfulness exercises to find peace amidst the chaos.

Chapter Nine

The Role of Support Systems

> "Alone we can do so little; together we can do so much."
> —Helen Keller

As you embark on the journey as collegiate aviation students, you must recognize that flying solo is not the path to success. In the dynamic world of aviation, having a robust support system is invaluable as you navigate your training and beyond. This chapter delves into the significance of mentorship, coaching, peer support, and the importance of seeking professional help when needed. Together, these pillars form the bedrock of a thriving aviation career.

Highlighting the Importance of Support Systems

Aviation is a challenging and rewarding endeavor that demands continuous growth and development. Mentorship emerges as a beacon of wisdom, proving us with valuable insights and guidance from experienced aviators who have walked the path before us. A mentor's wisdom can prove invaluable, enabling us to navigate through uncharted territories and emerge stronger and more confident.

Senior coaching/advisors on the other hand is like having a friendly chat with yourself, where coaches dig into what you already know deep down. It's like opening a treasure chest of your insights and skills, revealing not just what's right for you but also totally doable in your own special way.

It's a bit like a self-discovery journey, helping you find the hidden strengths and wisdom you've had all along, steering you towards a path where success feels not just real but completely within.

Notes:

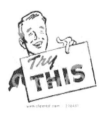

How to Ask a Mentor to Be Your Mentor:

Identify Potential Mentors: Look for individuals in the aviation field whose experience, expertise, and values align with your goals and aspirations. They should be someone you respect and admire for their achievements and character.

Build a Relationship: Before formally asking someone to be your mentor, take the time to build a relationship with them. Attend aviation events, conferences, or training sessions where you might meet potential mentors. Engage in conversations, ask questions, and express genuine interesting their insights.

Express Your Intentions: When you feel comfortable and have established rapport, express your interest in mentorship. Let them know that you admire their work and would greatly appreciate their guidance as you progress in your aviation career.

Articulate Your Goals: Be clear about your career goals and what you hope to achieve through mentorship. Share your aspirations and the areas in which you believe their mentorship could be particularly beneficial.

Ask for Their Guidance: Once you've expressed your intentions and goals, ask if they would be willing to serve as your mentor. Use polite and respectful language, such as, "Would you consider being my mentor as I pursue my aviation career?"

Be Open to Their Response: Understand that not everyone you approach will be available or willing to take on a mentoring role. Be gracious and respectful of their decision, whether it's a yes or no. If they decline, don't take it personally; they may have other commitments or reasons.

Set Expectations: If they agree to be your mentor, discuss and set clear expectations for how mentorship relationship will work. This includes the frequency of meetings, preferred communication methods, and any specific areas of focus.

Express Gratitude: Always express your gratitude for their willingness to mentor you.

Recognize that their time and guidance are valuable and be sure to acknowledge their contribution to your growth and development.

Remember that mentorship or coaching is a two-way street. While your mentor/coach will provide guidance and support, you should also be proactive in seeking their advice, acting on their feedback, and demonstrating your commitment to your own growth. A strong mentorship/coaching relationship can significantly contribute to your success in the aviation field.

Various Avenues to Find a Coach in Aviation:

Professional Coaching Services:

Seek specialized coaching services for aviation career development or personal growth. These platforms connect individuals with certified coaches experienced in aviation, providing structured guidance and support aligned with your goals.

Aviation Coaching Programs:

Look into coaching programs offered by aviation organizations or training institutions.

These programs, featuring one-on-one sessions or workshops, are led by experienced coaches focusing on skill development, goal setting, and overcoming challenges.

Online Platforms for Professional Coaches:

Utilize online platforms like the International Coach Federation (ICF) or coaching directories to find certified coaches with aviation expertise. These coaches offer personalized sessions tailored to your needs, be it career guidance, skill enhancement, or overcoming specific challenges.

When selecting a coach, clearly define your objectives, ensuring they match the coach's expertise. Effective coaching involves a collaborative relationship where the coach guides you to discover solutions and achieve your goals through thoughtful questioning and feedback.

Encouraging Seeking Professional Help

In the quest for excellence, you must also recognize that seeking professional help when needed is a testament to strength and resilience. Mental wellness is as vital as technical skills, and there may be moments when you face challenges that require professional support.

Engage with aviation mental health professionals (I can provide you with a list) who offer safe spaces for you to explore your thoughts and emotions and address any hurdles that may arise in your aviation journey. Their expertise equips you with coping mechanisms, strategies for stress management, and tools to maintain mental clarity in high-pressure situations, and sensitive to the unique airline industry. By seeking trusted professional help, you reinforce your commitment to being the best pilot you can be and prioritize your overall well-being, and not only your safety but everyone's safety.

Conclusion

Incorporating self-awareness and mindfulness into your lives lays the foundation for a fulfilling and successful aviation career. However, to truly thrive, you must recognize the significance of building a robust support system.

Mentors serve as beacons of knowledge, guiding you through the skies with their wisdom and experience. Coaching brings out the best in you. Embracing peer support creates an aviation community bonded by shared dreams and challenges. Together, uplift and empower one another to reach new heights.

As we navigate the skies and continue to explore the vast horizon of aviation, let us cherish and nurture our support systems. Together, we forge a community of aviators united in camaraderie and growth, enriching our lives and the skies we soar. If you have any questions, thoughts, or experiences to share, I encourage you to do so, fostering a dialogue that empowers us all on our path to success as collegiate aviators.

Chapter Ten

Q&A Session

> "In the sky, there is no distinction
> of east and west. People create
> distinctions out of their own minds,
> and then believe them to be true."
> —Gautama Buddha

As we near the end of our journey through the world of aviation, it's time for an open and interactive Q&A session. This is your opportunity to seek clarity, share insights, and explore any topics related to mental health in aviation, building resilience, or anything else we've discussed.

Question and Answer Bank

Student A: How can I effectively manage stress during intense flight training?

Captain O: Managing stress during flight training is crucial for your well-being and performance. Consider implementing mindfulness techniques, such as deep breathing exercises and visualization, to stay focused and centered in high-pressure situations. Additionally, prioritize self-care, engage in activities that relax and rejuvenate you.

- **Student B: How can I overcome imposter syndrome and gain confidence in my abilities as a future pilot?**

- **Captain O:** Imposter syndrome is common among aspiring aviators and professionals alike. Remember that it's normal to feel self-doubt, especially when taking on new challenges. Celebrate your achievements, no matter how small, and recognize that every pilot faces a learning curve. Let go of perfectionism, that's a myth. There is not "perfect" anything ... it's all about perception. Cultivate self-compassion, share your failures, and accept it and learn from it.

- **Student C: How can we maintain a work-life balance during rigorous flight training?**

- **Captain O:** Balancing flight training with other aspects of life is essential for overall well-being. Stay focused. You'll only have to do this for a short amount of time in comparison to your entire life. Set realistic and achievable goals, allowing time for personal activities outside of aviation. Going for a walk comes to mind. Communicate with your instructors and peers about your needs and limitations. Remember that taking breaks and engaging in "down time" are not distractions but essential for staying renewed, refreshed, and motivated.

- **Student D: What are some effective coping strategies for managing anxiety during flights?**

- **Captain O:** Anxiety is a natural response to challenging situations, some of us have more than other, but it can be managed effectively. Practice mindfulness techniques to stay present and reduce anxious thoughts. Engage in pre-flight mental preparation, reviewing SOP procedures and potential scenarios to boost confidence. It's difficult to study everything. Seek support from instructors and peers and remember that it's okay to take a moment to gather yourself before proceeding. And my number one answer is – sleep is your superpower. I talk about this more extensively in my book.

- **Student E: How can I develop a growth mindset in my aviation career?**

- **Captain O:** Developing a growth mindset is crucial for embracing challenges and continuous improvement in life and on the flight deck. Embrace failures and setbacks as opportunities for growth and learning. Stay curious and open to feedback, and view challenges as stepping-stones toward improvement. Recognize that every experience, whether positive or negative, contributes to your development as a pilot.

- **Student F: What strategies have you found effective in overcoming gender-related challenges or biases within the male-dominated industry?**

- **Captain O:** I have found 3 key strategies effective in overcoming gender-related challenges and biases:

- **Advocate for yourself:** Don't be afraid to advocate for your career advancement, fair compensation and equal opportunities. Even though, typically seniority drives equal opportunities not all of you will seek out the skies as a career.

- **Network:** Build a strong network of supportive colleagues, both male and female. Seek out one senior trustworthy "listening partner" who can provide coaching/mentoring based on their real-world relatable experiences.

- **Professionalism:** Maintain the highest level of professionalism in your interactions with colleagues, superiors, and subordinates. Your professionalism will speak for itself and help combat any stereotypes or biases.

Summarizing Key Takeaways

Throughout our journey, we have explored the importance of health and mental wellness in aviation, building resilience, and seeking support systems. Emphasizing self-awareness and mindfulness has proven to enhance decision-making and overall well-being in the cockpit.

Remember that you are not alone on this aviation adventure. Embrace mentorship/coaching and peer support to foster camaraderie and share insights. Seek professional help when needed, as it reflects your commitment to prioritizing mental well-being.

As collegiate aviators, prioritize self-care and work-life balance, as they are essential components of building resilience. Embrace challenges with a growth mindset, recognizing that every experience contributes to your growth as a pilot.

By taking these key takeaways to heart, you set the foundation for a successful and fulfilling aviation career. Continue to explore and learn, support one another, and let your passion for aviation soar to new heights. Safe flights and blue skies ahead!

Chapter Eleven

Making Mental Health a Priority in Aviation

Throughout this book, we have explored essential topics that are fundamental to your success as aspiring aviators.

The Significance of Mental Health in Aviation

We began our exploration by understanding the significance of mental health in aviation.

We learned how our mental well-being directly influences our performance, decision-making, and overall safety in the cockpit. By prioritizing our mental health, we lay the groundwork for a successful and fulfilling aviation career.

Building Resilience Through Self-Awareness and Mindfulness

Next, we delved into the powerful tools of self-awareness and mindfulness.

Building mental resilience is crucial for navigating challenges with clarity and focus.

By understanding our emotions, thoughts, and actions and staying fully present in the moment, we can make informed decisions and forge a deeper connection to the flight experience.

Creating a Healthier Cockpit Environment

We explored the importance of teamwork, communication, and support systems in creating a healthier cockpit environment.

Emphasizing open dialogue and seeking support when needed fosters a culture of understanding and compassion within the aviation community.

Remember, seeking professional help is not a sign of weakness but a strength that demonstrates our commitment to being the best pilots we can be.

Fostering Mental Well-Being in Aviation

In conclusion, I extend my heartfelt gratitude to each of you for your time and engagement during this presentation.

Your dedication to learning and growing as aspiring aviators is truly commendable.

I encourage you to carry forward the dialogue on mental health in aviation within your circles and the wider aviation community.

Embrace a Mindful Journey in Aviation

As you continue your journey in aviation, I urge you to embrace self-awareness, mindfulness, and the support of your peers and mentors.

Prioritize your mental well-being as you navigate the skies, for it is the foundation on which success is built.

Stay Connected and Informed

Should you have any further inquiries or wish to discuss any aspect further, please feel free to reach out to me at reyne@piloting2wellbeing.com.

I am here to support and guide you on your aviation path.

Recommended Resources

Additionally, I have compiled a list of recommended resources related to mental health in aviation.

These include books, articles, and organizations that offer valuable insights and support.

Embrace these resources to deepen your understanding and commitment to mental well-being.

A Final Call to Action

As we part ways today, my final call to action for each of you is to make mental health a priority in your aviation journey.

Remember that you are not alone; we are a community that supports and uplifts one another.

Let's continue fostering a culture of mental health awareness, resilience, and compassion in aviation.

Fly High and Keep Reaching for the Skies!

Thank you once again for your unwavering dedication. Fly high, take care, and keep reaching for the skies!

Together, we can create a safer, more supportive, and successful future for ourselves and the aviation industry.

**Blue Skies and Safe Flights Always,
Reyné O'Shaughnessy**

Book Reyné O'Shaughnessy as your Keynote Speaker and You're Guaranteed to Make Your Event Inspirational, Motivational, Highly Entertaining and Unforgettable!

Captain Reyné O'Shaughnessy (Ret.) has been a commercial airline pilot for over 34 years for a Fortune 50 company. She has logged over 10,000 hours of total heavy jet flight time. Her aircraft experience includes B727, B757/B767, Airbus 300/310, and notably, thirty four years ago she was one of the first women B747 qualified.

As the Founder of Piloting 2 Wellbeing, Reyné proudly partners with global solutions-oriented organizations that are serious about well-being and good health.

As a speaker, she especially enjoys connecting with audiences who have a desire to increase their own wellbeing, address the challenges of high-pressure careers, or decrease stress within their personal and professional lives..

Her unique style inspires, empowers and entertains audiences while giving them the tools and strategies they need and want to build and grow successful sustainable brands and businesses and become The Authority.

For more information and to book Reyné for your next event, visit www.Piloting2Wellbeing.com/Contact

Made in the USA
Middletown, DE
13 January 2024